Sex,
Prostate Cancer
& Me

ISBN-10: 1466221704
EAN-13: 9781466221703
Library of Congress 1-369464051
CreateSpace, North Charleston, SC
PRINTED IN THE UNITED STATES OF AMERICA

M. J. McDowell's

Sex, Prostate Cancer & Me

—II—

A WIFE'S CHRONICLE
OF HER HUSBAND'S PROSTATE CANCER,
DIAGNOSIS, RADICAL PROSTATECTOMY
&
SEXUAL RECOVERY

THIS BOOK IS DEDICATED TO
MY HUSBAND & SON

CONTENTS

PREFACE

Prostate cancer represents the second high-est cancer death rate for men. It is estimat-ed that in 2010, approximately 217,730[1] men in the U.S. will be diagnosed with prostate cancer and approximately 32,050[2] will die. Those who survive will find their lives forever changed.

Prostate cancer does not discriminate based on socioeconomic standing or religion; whether you are gay or straight, married or single. However, there are categories that place certain men in higher risk categories[3] than others. Regardless of how, why or when someone is diagnosed with prostate cancer, everyone shares the same emotion. Fear.

Fear of death. Fear of impotence.

---

1 http://www.cancer.gov/cancertopics/types/prostate
2 http://www.cancer.gov/cancertopics/types/prostate
3 See Page 60 "high risk categories"

————————

My name is M.J. McDowell. My husband and I shared those fears. This is my chronicle of overcoming fears, obstacles and finding a way not merely to cope, but to prevail.

At the time of my husband Gerry's diagnosis of prostate cancer I was 46 years old and Gerry was 56. This is my story of how we conquered the challenges of prostate cancer.

When Gerry was diagnosed with prostate cancer, the first thing I did was scour the Internet, the local library and book stores for information regarding the choices for treatment and the implications of each choice for my husband. While my immediate concern was Gerry's survival, nothing I read addressed my second concern, the impact on our sex life. Nothing I found addressed the topic of sex in any useful manner. My husband and I are young enough that sex remains a mutually satisfying and important part of our relationship. Motivated by my frustration, I decided to try to assist others that might have the same concern.

We-and I will use the term often because this has been a journey travelled together, are now 5 years beyond Gerry's radical prostatectomy surgery and time has provided me the advantage of perspective and evaluation. It is my intent to speak frankly about the most intimate particulars of our experiences, beginning with the diagnosis, decision to remove the prostate, recovery from surgery and ending with the details of adjustments to our sex life, post-surgery. This experience has encouraged us to grow, both sexually and as a couple and I want to encourage others to be proactive.

Gerry and I are a case in point that quality of life can improve after prostate cancer treatment if challenges are met with an open mind and perseverance.

I met Gerry when as a young woman I was hired by the company he owned. Gerry was ten years older than me, mature, experienced, raised in a major metropolitan environment by professional and thoroughly modern parents. I was raised in a more rural setting, sheltered by protective parents and a small religious community. My childhood and that of my brothers and sisters were regulated by strict religious practices and we were discouraged from socializing with our more "worldly" neighbors. Regardless of our different backgrounds, Gerry and I were undeniably attracted to one another. We were seriously dating within a year. It was not long before we were completely inseparable, totally smitten. I knew with absolute certainty that Gerry was a man I could love forever. Our years together have proven this to be true in ways that at the time I could not have imagined.

I have spent more than 25 years with Gerry, working side-by-side, operating a small business and raising a family. Sex has always been a joy for us. Our chemistry has been unfailingly good and our mutual attraction remains undiminished by time. When Gerry was diagnosed with prostate cancer, I remember thinking how unfair that we could potentially lose this aspect of our marriage that has never had a downside or required effort. I realize that the importance we place on intimacy in our relationship may be less than some folks or more than others, but intimacy has been a strong component in our partnership and we were both unwilling to accept its loss as an inevitable by-product of cancer treatment. We had, prior to prostate cancer, found time to include sex and romance in our daily lives.

Maintaining a healthy, happy, long-term relationship, without the challenge of a major illness requires attentiveness. For many couples, the additional stress of operating a small business would increase the potential for conflict. Fortunately, we have found just the opposite to be true. We found that our commitment to one another and the work ethic necessary to maintain a successful family business has been a positive influence and enhanced our ability to deal with the challenge of prostate cancer. Perhaps, because of business, Gerry and I have developed an appreciation for the crucial importance of discussing problems honestly, even when the topic is uncomfortable.

When I felt overwhelmed by the demands of Gerry's treatment and the demands of the business, our extended families pitched in. I cannot adequately express my gratitude for all the "little" things that were taken care by many helpful hands. The adjustment and treatment phases that follow a diagnosis of cancer are distressing and disruptive. A major illness presents an opportunity to reach out for and accept help from those who love you. They will feel better if you let them participate and it can be immeasurably helpful for you too, especially if there are children at home.

A diagnosis of prostate cancer changes your sex life. Regardless of your course of treatment, sex for you and your partner will require adjustments once treatment begins.

Gerry and I talked extensively throughout the process of diagnosis, our joint decision of treatment by radical prostatectomy, and the ongoing effect that it has had on our sex life and our marriage. I am not a medical professional and my simplification of medical terms commonly used with this diagnosis does not replace professional advice. I am simply laying out my understanding of what I have gathered from a wide variety of reading material and conversations with my husband's physicians over an extended time.

I continue to be astonished by the amount of couples that face this cancer in silence.

Following our disclosure of Gerry's diagnosis to friends and colleagues, we were surprised as one person after another came forward to express concern and to communicate their experiences with prostate cancer. We heard from family members as well as people with whom we encountered on a regular basis professionally. In all cases, we had no idea these individuals had been living with prostate cancer in apparent isolation.

What I quickly intuited is that this disease is a considered a very private matter. A diagnosis of prostate cancer inevitably involves issues of erections and sex; topics of intimacy that many people consider inherently private in nature. Because people are so hesitant to share their frustrations and challenges regarding sex, they are unintentionally isolating themselves, in essence, preventing or delaying a possible solution. To varying degrees, every couple that is affected by prostate cancer has obstacles to confront. We all engage in sex, but are not necessarily accustomed to discussing personal sexual practices in casual conversation.

If you and your partner are willing, there are creative ways to improve sex after treatment, as Gerry and I have discovered.

After Gerry's surgery, it became clear that spontaneous sex and "quickies" would have to be redefined. We found that we had to be much more structured to allow for new and necessary accommodations when making love. We discovered new techniques and positions through trial and error that have proven successful and dependable for us, and were fun during the learning process. I have shared some of those in the chapter about sex.

CHAPTER 1

PSA TEST

Following a routine exam at age 54, my husband Gerry's PSA[4] results registered an increased number from previous years. PSA, or prostate-specific-antigen is present in the blood stream and is measured by a blood test. Healthy men generally have a low PSA number. An increase of the PSA number can indicate an enlarged prostate or inflammation. An enlarged prostate is expected as men age, but routine testing will give physicians a baseline and allow them to determine if changes warrant additional testing.

Our family physician prudently referred Gerry to an Urologist for a consult and possible diagnostic prostate biopsy. The Urologist reviewed Gerry's labs and asked questions about his family history. Based on the combination

---

4 See Page 59

of a year-on-year PSA elevation and his family history a biopsy to confirm or eliminate cancer was recommended..

The diagnostic process would begin with a surgical biopsy, followed by an office visit to review those results. If the biopsy results proved positive, the doctor would recommend a course of treatment and explain Gerry's options.

There is controversy regarding the value of PSA testing and the early detection of prostate cancer. There is a clear dispute between the insurance industry, reflecting new government recommendations, and the medical community. There are also suggestions that unnecessary intervention or overreaction to a diagnosis of prostate cancer that may be irrelevant (too slow growing or a type that is not sufficiently aggressive) results in functional damage, when the cancer left alone would not be fatal. Accordingly, there is an argument for cost cutting by doing away with annual PSA screening.

The undisputed fact is that prostate cancer is the second highest cause of cancer deaths for men in the United States. The medical community argues that early detection and appropriate treatment can eradicate beginning stage cancer and prolong and improve quality of life for more advanced cases. I remain immensely grateful to the doctors directly involved in Gerry's care for both the early detection and life saving treatment that he received.

CHAPTER 2

GERRY'S FAMILY HISTORY

When we received notice that Gerry's PSA numbers were elevated, our thoughts turned to Gerry's dad. We knew that because Gerry's dad had succumbed to prostate cancer, there existed family history that placed Gerry in a high-risk category for the disease. Knowing that the propensity existed-and being presented with personally facing cancer are two different realities. One is an academic concept; the other involves the unpredictable aspect of emotional involvement.

We couldn't prevent our minds from replaying Gerry's dad, Abe's, last years over and over, like an old and well remembered film.

At the time of Abe's diagnosis in the early 1970's, PSA tests were not in use. The first symptom that Abe experienced was difficulty urinating. His initial exam resulted in a diagnosis of, and treatment for, an enlarged prostate, a common malady.

Trained as a physician and surgeon, Abe was accustomed to making difficult decisions. As a WWII trauma surgeon, he had to make life and death decisions every day, decide whether amputations were necessary to preserve life, whether a soldiers' wounds were terminal or treatable. He loved the pace of trauma surgery, but the loss of life and limb took its toll on him.

Upon his return from WWII, Abe chose to specialize in the field of obstetrics/gynecology. He spent well over thirty years delivering babies and caring for women. He remained a skilled and sought after surgeon, dedicated and thorough, one of the first physicians to perform lumpectomy instead of total mastectomy whenever possible.

As his prostate symptoms continued to worsen, rather than abate, Abe realized that he was probably dealing with a more serious matter than simply an enlarged prostate. More tests were performed and a diagnosis of prostate cancer was confirmed.

Treatment choices were limited at that time and Abe's cancer was very aggressive. Together, Abe and his urologist decided that, although radical, the best option to slow and potentially stop the cancer from spreading was surgical castration. Today, there are pharmaceuticals that can be administered to control the production of testosterone and retard the growth of cancer within the prostate.

Castration was an extreme option and a difficult decision for him to make. He did not divulge any of what he was struggling through with his family and friends until after the surgery. I think he was afraid we might talk him out of it.

Abe had just entered his 7th decade at the time of his surgery, born in 1906, at the beginning of the century; he was by all accounts still vital. He was an extraordinary man, stubborn, frighteningly intelligent, vigorous and energetic. He was the type of person that ran, rather than walked, napped rather than slept. His presence was felt whenever he entered a room. He was not ready to die. He understood more fully than most of us the consequences of his decision, and he was prepared to live with those consequences.

Abe had the surgery. He was tenacious, driving 400 miles to visit Gerry and I immediately after his surgery, catheter still in place. During his stay, he insisted on lengthy daily walks. Not once did I have reason to question his health. This particular visit followed the same pattern as previous stays.

It was only after he returned to his home, following his stay with us, that he disclosed the cancer diagnosis, his choice of treatment by castration, and the fact that he was just out of the hospital following surgery when he came to visit with us. We were stunned and could not comprehend why he had not confided in us earlier.

Gerry and I both felt that it would have been beneficial to all if he had allowed family the opportunity to provide support, encouragement and love. It must have been a frightening ordeal to go through alone. Abe said he felt that the surgery was necessary and he had not wanted us to worry.

Following Abe's disclosure, our family circled the wagons. Abe's ex-wife, Gerry's mother, still resided in the same city as Abe, and was willing and able to accompany him to doctor appointments and make sure that he was taking good care of himself. Abe also had several close friends, who along with his ex-wife were close enough in proximity to have regular involvement in his care and wellbeing. Gerry and I traveled to visit often. We were as actively involved in his continued care as he would allow.

In a very short time period, it was determined that Abe's cancer had metastasized. He was given six months to live.

Abe survived for almost seven years. I attribute those seven years to his strength of character. For the first five years, he continued to work and enjoyed a more limited (non-sexual), but satisfying social life. He was productive and independent.

In the sixth year following surgery, the spreading cancer began to sap his energy.

It became difficult for him to complete tasks necessary for daily life. Abe agreed to sell his home and move in with Gerry and I. He was realistic about his health and chose to spend his remaining time with us. We had discussed his wishes and would honor his choices.

The first year spent with us was enjoyable. Even though cancer had invaded Abe's spine, stomach and bones, he had no complaints of pain or discomfort, but he tired easily. He would come in to town almost every working day and have lunch with Gerry, a business colleague and myself. Abe's appetite was voracious and although he ate everything he could get his hands on, his weight slid inexorably downward and we knew that our time together, though precious, was limited. I treasure the memories of that year.

Abe's final year was not so pleasant. As the cancer invaded his spine, steadily creeping upwards, eventually reaching his brain, Abe began having mini-strokes. Fortunately, his finances allowed us to hire nurses, which permitted him to remain at home with round-the-clock medical care.

Serendipity provided us with Malena, a tiny, plucky, multilingual nurse who took her job as Abe's caregiver very seriously. An effect of Abe's mini-strokes was for him to speak in a mix of German, Polish, English and Yiddish. Gerry and I had difficulty with the mix of languages and communication became frustrating for us. Not Malena-she was thrilled. She was fluent in German and understood his Yiddish too. Caring for Abe allowed her to speak her native tongue. When she discovered how much he relished her German cooking, she spoiled him with dishes from his childhood.

Abe had emigrated as a youngster in 1910 from Poland. Gerry's mother was Austrian, and German was the private language used by Gerry's parents when he was a boy. Neither Gerry, nor I spoke German, so it was our good fortune to have hired someone able to comfort Abe in the language of his childhood.

Home became a medical ward. There was a hospital bed, various apparatus', appliances, pills, and bedpans with accompanying odors that lingered, regardless of constant and thorough cleaning.

Abe's world had become increasingly smaller, shrinking to within the walls of the house. He still had preferences and directed the household accordingly. He became obsessed with CNN. He was enthralled by access to 24/7, worldwide news coverage. In the late 1970's cable stations were limited, no one had personal computers, there was no public Internet access.

The time came when the effect of multiple strokes made it impossible for Abe to communicate in any language. Very shortly after communication became impossible, his body began to fail. Abe's last months were spent in and out of the hospital. Abe died just a few days shy of his seventy-ninth birthday.

Caring for Abe at the end of his life greatly influenced our decision to treat Gerry's cancer by radical prostatectomy. We had watched the disease's natural progression in a very personal way. If possible, Gerry would not follow the same prostate cancer path of his father.

CHAPTER 3

BIOPSY

Prostate biopsy can be performed at the doctor's facility or in a hospital. Gerry's biopsy was performed in a hospital under general anesthesia. Gerry and I met the surgeon who performed the biopsy, Dr. Young, for the first time just prior to sedation. He wanted to confirm that we understood why we were there and to explain the biopsy procedure to us. Dr. Young began by reviewing the process of sedation and it's risks. He then carefully explained the methods he would employ during the procedure itself.

Dr. Young expressed his personal preference for taking samples from multiple sites of the prostate. I do not know if there is a medical standard regarding the number of samples taken or a suggested pattern of biopsy samples. I do know that the first Urologist we saw suggested there would be 8 samples taken. Dr. Young explained that he would take 12 to 16 samples from random sites around the perimeter of the prostate. I have been told that it is not unusual to have to go through the biopsy process several times before the part of the prostate that has cancer cells is discovered.

Dr. Young's rationale for the larger number of samples was that if a cancer is in its beginning stage; the odds of identifying and locating it increase exponentially with each additional extraction. If the cancer is aggressive, a liberal sampling could mean the difference of life and death.

I felt comfort knowing the odds for discovering a cancer before it has escaped the prostate gland were in our favor because of Dr. Young's personal philosophy. We were told that the procedure involves lab processing and interpretation and that it could take 5-10 days before the pathology report would become available. We were scheduled to meet with the primary urologist about two weeks after the biopsy to review the results.

Once the samples are taken, they are sent to a pathologist, a doctor who specializes in examining blood and tissue samples under a microscope. Upon completion of the testing, the pathologist prepares a formal written report that is sent to the requesting physician, at which time the results can be given to the patient.

I firmly believe that it is in the patient's best interest to request a copy of all test results and to make sure that every doctor participating is given a copy. It's also a good idea to maintain a personal file with all accumulated data.

CHAPTER 4

DIAGNOSIS

On the day of our appointment following Gerry's biopsy, we were ushered into a consultation room, nervously anticipating a review of the biopsy findings.

That meeting is imprinted with absolute clarity in my mind. There is one urology practice in our town and it occupies a modern building the size of a small hospital with facilities, equipment and staff to perform almost any procedure. This particular practice did not administer general anesthesia in their office at the time of Gerry's biopsy, but practices in other locations may.

Based on our experience, this particular urology practice followed an assembly-line process that streamlined workflow but was not sensitive to the patient.

The room we were brought to was located on an upper floor, at the end of a very long hall. Entry was through a narrow door. The room was Spartan: It had the look and feel of a hastily re-purposed closet-a tiny, austere space, maybe 8-10 feet square, and the only light source, a dim ceiling fixture. There were two door-the one we used for entry from the hall and a second door that permitted entry from an interior office. The furnishings were glaringly sparse in comparison to the opulence of the waiting rooms and other office and exam rooms we had previously experienced. The room was filled to capacity by a small, round, plain wood table with four wooden chairs and unadorned walls. No brochures, no magazines, not even a box of tissues or a trash can. It's funny how the mind preserves the smallest details when life-altering moments are recalled. An unfamiliar doctor arrived, introduced himself by saying, "Hello, I'm Dr. Jackson and I am the doctor that will be performing your radical prostatectomy surgery[5]. Do you have questions before I explain the procedure to you?"

Immediately I experienced a horrible sinking sensation, a cold, hard fist clamped deep within my belly, squeezing out my breath and causing me to bend over in physical pain. Radical prostatectomy? Cancer? Yes, I had known that it was a possibility, but in my heart I was unprepared for a definitive diagnosis of cancer.

---

5 See page 19

Gerry was young, fit; active-his sex drive was strong. Based on our past experiences with Abe, I expected there to be signs of impending trouble: difficulty urinating, difficulties with sexual performance, perhaps tiredness or weakness. I didn't really know, I just thought there should be some physical manifestation. Of course, now I know better. Prostate cancer can be silent-it can be both silent and deadly.

In my mind, Gerry did not fit the profile of a cancer victim that I had envisioned. I believed at the time that if someone had an illness as serious as cancer that surely there would be signs, symptoms, some indicator of trouble on the horizon. I was stunned. So was Gerry. We both gazed at Dr. Jackson, stupefied.

Based on our reaction, Dr. Jackson immediately realized that a step had been missed. Apparently, the scheduling department completely sidestepped our meeting with the primary urologist to discuss the outcome of the biopsy. They had instead scheduled us directly with Dr. Jackson, a urological surgeon. He had expected to consult an informed patient who had already chosen a surgical path for treatment. Instead he found himself confronted with a couple that had not been told that the diagnosis was indeed cancer.

What a shock for all of us. Fortunately, Dr. Jackson was a patient and kind man. After Gerry and I regained our composure, Dr. Jackson explained the biopsy results, reviewed the options and consequences, answered questions and clarified definitions of unfamiliar terminology.

We asked Dr. Jackson to give us a breakdown of the report. He flipped over a document and proceeded to draw a diagram[6] of Gerry's anatomy to explain his recommendation in favor of a radical prostatectomy. In Gerry's case, the cancer was positioned in a small, tightly spaced grouping that could have easily been missed by a surgeon with a preference for less biopsy samples. Dr. Jackson explained that according to Gerry's Gleason Score[7] he believed that radical prostatectomy surgery could successfully eradicate Gerry's cancer.

Gerry's Gleason Score indicated that the cancer cells biopsied were moderately aggressive. Dr. Jackson explained that because the diagnosis was made early, the odds were greatly in our favor that the cancer was contained within the prostate gland. Removal of the prostate should then remove the cancer and its source. Dr. Jackson suggested that we consider seeking a second opinion before making a treatment decision. He wanted us to be completely certain and committed to the course of treatment chosen.

---

6 SEE PAGE 42
7 SEE PAGE 57

Using Gerry's Gleason Score of 3+3=6, Dr. Jackson gave us a run-down of the following treatment options to treat Gerry's cancer.

Note: This list may not be current. It reflects the options available to Gerry and I at the time we made our decision to have radical prostatectomy surgery.

1. Brachytherapy, commonly called "seed therapy"-radiation is placed within or as close to the cancer cells as possible

2. Cryotherapy-minimally invasive surgery with the goal of killing the cancer by freezing it with extreme cold

3. Hormone Therapy-used to lower PSA by slowing cancer growth

4. Radiation-has the potential to cure some cancers and is used as part of the treatment plan for more advanced cancers-it has the potential to shrink existing cancerous tumors or to slow their growth and prolong life

5. Radical Prostatectomy-the most radical treatment that completely removes the prostate-this surgery can be performed using one of two methods: one; conventional surgery through the abdomen, or two; a less invasive technique, utilizing the da Vinci® robotic tool

———

Prostate cancer treatments require patients to be monitored for an extended time through prostate-specific antigen (PSA) tests. The doctor managing treatment of the prostate cancer determines the PSA testing schedule.

When Dr. Jackson felt confident that Gerry and I had grasped the options laid out, he excused himself, telling us that we could use the room as long as we needed. We did not stay. Gerry and I headed out to the car, our minds reeling with all that we had absorbed. We traveled in silence on the parkway for about 45 minutes, grateful for the distraction of passing scenery and the comfort of familiar sights and the sound of passing traffic. As we approached the exit for our office, we agreed to finish out the workday and wait until the evening before trying to talk things out. We both needed time to process the barrage of thoughts now running rampant through our minds.

Later, at home, I confessed my fears to Gerry. I did not want him to die. I wanted him to live and grow old with me. I was afraid that he might not consider a treatment as radical as a prostatectomy. To say that I was conflicted about the choices and consequences presented would be a gross understatement. I was leaning heavily in favor of radical prostatectomy surgery, yet I had concerns about

Gerry's quality-of-life if he did choose surgery. Both impotence and urinary incontinence are probable permanent conditions following any therapy for prostate cancer and Gerry and I know men who live with those complications, including an uncle, whose prostatectomy left him both impotent and incontinent.

My uncle Marion is the father of nine children, very active, a world traveler. His prostatectomy left him both impotent and incontinent. When the determination was made that he would not regain urinary continence, he chose to have a surgical device implanted in his penis to control the flow of urine. I don't know all of the details, but my aunt told me that there is a valve that Uncle Marion must open and close to release or stop the flow of urine. She said that he is supposed to perform this procedure every couple of hours throughout the day and that their travel destinations are now limited based on Uncle Marion's physical constraints. She said that because there is a foreign body in his penis, there is always a considerable risk of infection and he must adhere to a scrupulously clean hygiene regimen in order to avoid infection.

My head was reeling with all sorts of conflicting and meandering thoughts. I decided that the most sensible thing was to sit down with Gerry, list the pluses and minuses, then decide on a treatment and form an action plan.

Ironically, our neighbor Carl, 15 years Gerry's senior, was diagnosed with prostate cancer just a week following Gerry's diagnosis. Unfortunately, his cancer was too advanced for a radical prostatectomy or radiation cure. Carl's urologist gave him a life expectancy estimate of 6 months to 2 years. However, after consulting a urology oncologist, Carl was told that with an assortment of therapies he could expect to live 5 to 10 years. His oncologist used hormone therapy, radiation and chemotherapy to retard the cancer's advancement for as long as possible.

Both Carl and his wife wanted to continue treatment as long as Carl's quality of life remained satisfactory. He experienced ups and downs from the various treatments, including fatigue, impotence, hair loss, and nausea. Throughout the aggressive and continuous treatments, Carl maintained a positive attitude, said that he felt "pretty good" most of the time-experienced some physical weakness, but was able to get out and about and enjoy himself in a way that was satisfying to him.

Despite continuous treatment regimens, Carl's cancer spread to other areas of his body. Toward the end, his wife worried about a developing symptom of short-term memory loss, but it did not bother Carl, for obvious reasons and was not a quality-of-life problem. They were acutely aware that each day is a precious gift and did their utmost to make the most out of whatever time remained. Regardless of how upbeat the two of them were; I am reminded that Carl's diagnoses did not come early enough for a cure.

———

There is risk for both impotence and urinary incontinence from all prostate cancer treatments. Less invasive treatments only retard or slow the growth of cancer, it (treatment) must be monitored and managed permanently. Gerry and I agreed that the only reason not to choose a radical prostatectomy were if the cancer had broached the prostate gland. Regardless of the risk of impotence and incontinence, we still wanted to move forward with surgery. We have always been a strong, interdependent unit and were determined to grow old together.

Gerry and I have spent the greater portion of our lives practically joined at the hip. As partners in business and in life, we know each other well. We have spent all of our time together working towards common goals. We are extremely close and feel grateful for every day and are committed to continuing our life together.

CHAPTER 5

SURGERY

Surgery-the decision has been made to move forward with Gerry's radical prostatectomy. Before scheduling a day and time we wanted answers to several specific questions. With the prostate gone, what were Gerry's chances for an erection? Would we still be able to make love?

I requested success statistics from Dr. Jackson. He quoted his statistics, broken down by age. He boasted a "functional erection" success rate of 96% for men in my husband's age group. Dr. Jackson did caution us that even with those numbers, there was no guarantee, because every surgery and every person is unique.

We were told that post-surgery almost everyone experiences a temporary loss of bladder control and that for some it will be a permanent condition. The potential for Gerry spending the rest of his life in diapers was not appealing.

The same is true for a functional erection, even with the aid of drugs and appliances. Notice the word "functional". Viewed with hindsight, I would listen much more carefully for words that are used in conjunction with a qualifier and ask for clarification. Contemplating a future without sex worried both of us. We are inseparable. We work, live, play and love together. Gerry is my best friend and my lover. We are accustomed to regular, enthusiastic sex. I have never understood couples that complain about their partner's sexual appetite. For me, sex is like food. I am as passionately hungry for my husband as I am hungry for food. And I like to eat.

Cancer in any form just plain scares the hell out of anyone, but if you are fortunate enough to have an early diagnosis and the option to surgically remove the beast from your body, I cannot imagine opting not to do so.

Prostate cancer is still taboo in our society, much as breast cancer was a decade ago. However, today, we see pink ribbons for breast cancer awareness everywhere.

I have noticed cars sporting bumper stickers that say, "Save the Ta-Ta's", definitely a favorite of mine. I want to see prostate cancer given the same attention. Sex is important, but life is precious and with more than 240,000 new cases diagnosed annually in the United States, there are an overwhelming number of men, couples and families impacted by prostate cancer.

When interviewing surgeons, I urge the reader to ask their treating physician for his personal statistics. Ask for patient references, preferably from patients who are several years post-surgery and were in your age group at the time of their prostatectomy.

I feel strongly that working with a local doctor is prudent so that follow-up care is not compromised. Imagine compounding the difficulty of surgical complications with long distance travel.

The urology practice that we used offered a class to prepare us for the upcoming surgery. I would absolutely recommend attending such a class, if offered. The class that we attended was hosted by an experienced R.N. who was straightforward in explaining the physical procedure as well as what to expect during the hospital stay.

We were told to expect 3 to 6 hours for the surgery. The nurse said that someone from the surgical team would call the waiting room during the surgery to give updates. After the surgery's completion the surgeon would meet with the family to review the surgery and give them an estimate of expected hospital recovery time.

True to their word, a nurse provided updates by phone every hour during the surgery. Gerry's surgery took three and a half hours. Dr. Jackson came to the waiting area when it was over and said that Gerry's surgery had gone beautifully. He had not encountered any difficulties. Gerry's prostate was quite large, but Dr. Jackson said that he sees them in a range of sizes. He made note that he had been careful to; "leave the field wet". When I asked what he meant by that, he explained that a wet field meant that he had sutured loosely. This technique assists the nerves reattaching in a useful way. He told us that he anticipated Gerry's hospital stay at 3 to 5 days.

Dr. Jackson told me that the prostate had been sent to pathology to verify that the cancer was indeed contained. We received the pathology report during Gerry's hospital stay. The cancer cells were contained within the prostate; therefore, the surgery was successful.

A nurse explained that Gerry had a tube placed in his lower belly to drain fluids that accumulate in the abdomen after surgery. When the tube is removed it looks like a ragged hole. They literally poke a hole with the drain tube, so that when it is removed it looks like what it is-a puncture wound. The sight of Gerry's puncture was disconcerting to me, but it healed very quickly and today there is no scar at all. Gerry was one of the lucky guys whose tube was removed while in hospital, but about half will return home with the tube still in place and careful adherence to the care instructions are a must in order to prevent infection.

As the anesthesia wore off, Gerry experienced nausea. He was given medication to mitigate the nausea as soon as the staff became aware. Gerry realized that the nausea was an effect of intravenous narcotics for pain. He requested removal of the pain meds and the duty nurse got permission from the doctor to allow them to stop the drip delivery of narcotics. The nausea subsided. Unfortunately, as the nausea subsided, he was hit with a migraine. If there are medications that a person takes apart from the hospital, there are ways to preload the patients chart to allow them. Migraine Headaches! We had not planned for that occurrence and many hours passed before the doctor-on-call granted permission for Gerry to be given appropriate medication for his migraine.

We were told to expect the scrotum to be swollen, sore and bruised. A radical prostatectomy is major abdominal surgery and pain medication is de rigueur. Gerry was given extra strength Tylenol for the remainder of his stay. He has always had a high pain tolerance and was able to finish out the stay without the use of narcotics. In hospital, a number system of 1-10 is used to determine your level of pain and medication is dispensed accordingly.

Compression stockings are used to prevent blood clots that could cause stroke or death. The nurses caring for Gerry were not careful with these stockings and I found myself adjusting them constantly, they persistently bunched around his lower legs. Fortunately, we had been shown how to adjust the compression stockings in the pre-surgery class and knew that they must fit smoothly, without wrinkles in order to be effective.

It is important for the patient to enlist someone to undertake the role of advocate while in hospital. Nurses today are grossly overworked. It is up to the partner or advocate to ensure that the patient is getting appropriate care for his needs. Nurses do not have the authority to change patient orders on their own and they are often discouraged from disturbing doctors after regular hours. Try not to blame the nurses for the things they have no control over.

Hospital nursing schedules are tightly regulated. The lack of available one-on-one time is as frustrating for them as it is for the patient. A partner or advocate can be indispensible to helping the patient satisfy the requirements necessary for discharge. Nurses do not have time to help patients ambulate. Getting up and walking as much as possible is paramount to healing. Having someone to assist in this very important step cannot be understated. Just make sure to check with a duty nurse before undertaking any activity. There may be constraints or conditions that impact certain activities.

One of the hurdles all surgical patients must cross before discharge is to have a bowel movement. Anesthesia stops the normal movement of the intestinal tract and a bowel movement verifies that the patients' digestive system is functioning again.

CHAPTER 6

RECOVERY

The ancient hospital volunteer wheeled Gerry from his room to the car after first burying both he and the wheelchair precariously high with flowers, balloons and cards from well-wishers. At the car, we unloaded Gerry and carefully maneuvered him into the car, catheter still in place; drain tube removed at the last minute prior to his discharge. The tube/puncture wound was a bandaged, gaping and ragged hole. From naval to pubis a long line of metal staples ran the length of his belly. Please be mindful that there are internal stitches too and that most of the surgical work is not visible from the outside. Radical prostatectomy is major abdominal surgery.

I had prepared a nest for Gerry on our ground floor so that he could avoid stairs temporarily, have easy access to kitchen, bath and family, but he wanted to crawl into his own bed-upstairs. The stairs were a little tricky. If you've ever had your abdomen opened you will vividly recall how important those muscles are for achieving even the most basic movements. By hanging onto the railing and with some help from me he groped his way to the top and into bed. It was all I could do to get his shoes off before he fell into an exhausted asleep. While he rested I placed the various lotions, medicines and supplies within easy reach. I emptied the catheter bag and using a strip of cloth, knotted it loosely around the drain tube and tied it to the side of the bed. I was careful to leave enough wiggle room for Gerry to move without placing undue pressure on his penis.

The catheter goes home with almost every patient who has this surgery. Be prepared. The caretaker will have to diligently assist in caring for the site. The catheter required constant attention. It tugged and pulled at the head of his penis. The drain tube developed kinks and sharp bends that prevented proper draining.

I had to keep a log of Gerry's fluid output and watch for signs of fresh blood. There was quite a bit of brown in the urine, especially at first-no surprise considering the bleeding that was caused during surgery, but I was warned to keep a sharp eye out for "new blood".

Hydration is important. Clear urine is the indicator of adequate hydration.

The head of the penis at the insertion site must be kept scrupulously clean and antibacterial cream applied often to avoid infection, irritation and discomfort.

I found Gerry's after-surgery care both overwhelming and exhausting. I had prepared as much beforehand as I could; however my daily responsibilities of work, pet care, childcare, and groceries, cleaning and cooking still had to get done. Like a majority of folks out there, we did not have the financial resources to hire help, so while my days are normally very full, during Gerry's recovery every day presented new challenges. I needed to remind myself to be patient, gentle and loving and not let Gerry perceive how difficult the impact his surgery and recovery were for me.

Realistically, I knew that the load would soon lighten, but there were days when maintaining a happy face was an effort.

It helped to wake up each morning thankful for a fresh start and mindful that Gerry was just beginning recovery from major surgery and that he was free of prostate cancer. As exhausted as I was, I knew that he was tired, sore, not feeling very manly and sometimes frightened now that the surgery was over. I tried to focus on keeping his spirits up, encouraging him to become mobile as quickly as possible.

I would ask him to do simple things. "Honey, could you walk to the closet and grab a new pack of gauze?" Or, "I'm going to shower in 5 minutes, it would help me if you get in too. That way I can wash us both at the same time." It wasn't hard to motivate Gerry to get up and move around, but whether it is easy or hard, it must be done and the sooner the better.

After a couple of days in bed, Gerry became bored and managed, on his own, to strap the urine collection bag to his leg and ambulate around the house. A note; gentlemen, if you wear boxer shorts, you will want to invest in some tighty whities for this part of the surgical recovery. I bought Gerry's in a size smaller than usual and it was a great idea. Not only was everything from his abdomen to his penis incredibly tender, he still had the catheter attached. We were warned that the catheter is usually left in place for 10 to 20 days. We found that Gerry could pull on a pair tighty whities, add sweats, confident that the catheter was secure and unobtrusive enough to leave the house. He walked inside the house, around the yard, gingerly negotiating the neighborhood, using a cane for support. Gerry increased the length of his walks daily and his strength and mood improved accordingly.

We had previously been given instructions by the lecture-nurse to purchase a jumbo package of appropriately sized adult diapers from Sam's Club or Costco and we took several with us to the post-op appointment.

After checking the puncture and catheter sites, and palpitating Gerry's belly, Dr. Jackson asked Gerry if he wanted the catheter removed. Gerry immediately exclaimed, "Hell yes, take this thing out!" The doc called in his nurse to remove it.

Dr. Jackson's nurse used sterile water to expand a balloon inside the bladder to keep the catheter from coming out. Next, she flushed the catheter with sterile water, and then she drained the balloon. Last, she had him sit in a semi-prone position, told him that he would feel a strong pinch and on the count of 3 pulled it swiftly out. It was not painful. Gerry said it just felt like a hard tug.

His penis immediately began a steady urine drip. Gerry quickly slipped into the waiting diaper. The doctor came back in and advised Gerry to continue to wear diapers for 6 to 8 weeks before trying to taper off, cautioning that diaper dependence can be a significant hindrance to regaining bladder control.

It took a couple of days for the tenderness at the tip of penis to fade away after removal of the catheter.

Dr. Jackson's weaning method began with Kegel exercises to regain bladder control. (Yes, the same exercise given to pregnant women for the same purpose. Performing this exercise is simple and it can be done anywhere. Kegel employs your pelvic muscles. The easiest way to find your pelvic muscle is during urination. When you are mid-stream, try to hold/stop the flow. The muscle used to stop the flow is the one necessary for Kegel. It is as simple as this: (tighten – release – tighten-release). The recommendation was to slowly work up to three sets of ten each time the exercise is performed to physically strengthen bladder control.

When he felt he had some bladder control, Gerry was ready for the next step; short outings minus the diaper. The idea is to go to a public place where there is ready access to a bathroom. Dr. Jackson felt that patients who had the physical capability of urinary continence would recover more quickly by placing themselves in situations where it is socially unacceptable to pee your pants. Mind over matter. Dr. Jackson warned Gerry that total bladder control was not to be immediately expected and long-term bladder control was not guaranteed, but based on Gerry's internal surgical outcome, he could see no physical reason for my husband not to overcome his current state of incontinence.

We found there was wisdom to his thinking. Gerry's body had to re-learn several functions all over again and he was game to try whatever it took.

We purchased a stay-dry mattress pad for nighttime damage control and at about the 2-3 week postoperative point Gerry returned to work for several hours at a time in diapers (that no one could see) and wearing sweat pants. Sweat pants are easy to get in to and out of, plus, they felt softer than trousers on his tender midsection.

While at work, Gerry remembered to practice Kegel at his desk, getting up and going to the toilet whenever he felt the slightest urge to urinate. Most of the time, getting there before the trickle began. The office was a friendly, supportive environment for Gerry as he worked to become fully functional.

It would be many months before Gerry became leak free. With the prostate removed, the stream of urine was significantly stronger. After urinating, no matter how much Gerry tried to shake his penis, it continued to dribble.

Another interesting note from this period is that Gerry found that whenever he moved his bowels the bladder released simultaneously as well. This occurs because the same muscle controls both the urethra and the rectum. It remains a predictable occurrence today. He learned very early on to tuck his penis between his knees when moving his bowels. Physical stress and sexual excitement caused urine to leak too.

A story. Gerry lifts weights. About eight weeks post surgery he was given the okay to begin normal activity... for him that included visiting the gym. I accompanied him as a precaution. I remember looking up from my bench when my peripheral vision caught a figure scurrying quickly past. It was Gerry. He returned a little while later and found me. He said that he was fine until he started to press real weight. He said that the moment he felt the full stress of the weights, his bladder began to dribble. He was worried that it would be obvious to others. Good thing he had a towel. Even better that he had urinated prior to beginning his work out so there wasn't much urine to spill.

For the next several weeks he used a menstrual pad while lifting weights. Lightweight and unobtrusive, maxi and mini-pads are extremely absorbent for their small size and are a good option for minor leaks. He eventually conquered the stress incontinence, but he still has to remember to relieve himself prior to undertaking strenuous activities. If he does something that requires really tensing the stomach muscles there is still a chance for minor leakage.

During those first weeks Gerry pushed himself to walk as much as possible every day. Initially, it was more like a daily hobble aided by a cane. At first he would begin enthusiastically and then; just as a young kitten or puppy, without warning his energy would suddenly evaporate and he would have to stop, sit and rest awhile before slowly continuing home. I firmly believe that Gerry's early attempts at physical activity helped to maintain his muscle tone and improved his ability to regain urinary continence.

It was about this time that Gerry began feeling horny again too. We took that as a good sign, because the doctor had told us that when a patient "feels something" than the nerves were still functional and the odds of achieving an erection and having sex were vastly improved. Conversely, there will be some men whose nerves do not reconnect and they will be impotent. If the desire is absent the frustration should be as well. The problems that occur are for the percentage of men who still desire sex, but are unable to perform.

MALE REPRODUCTIVE DRAWING

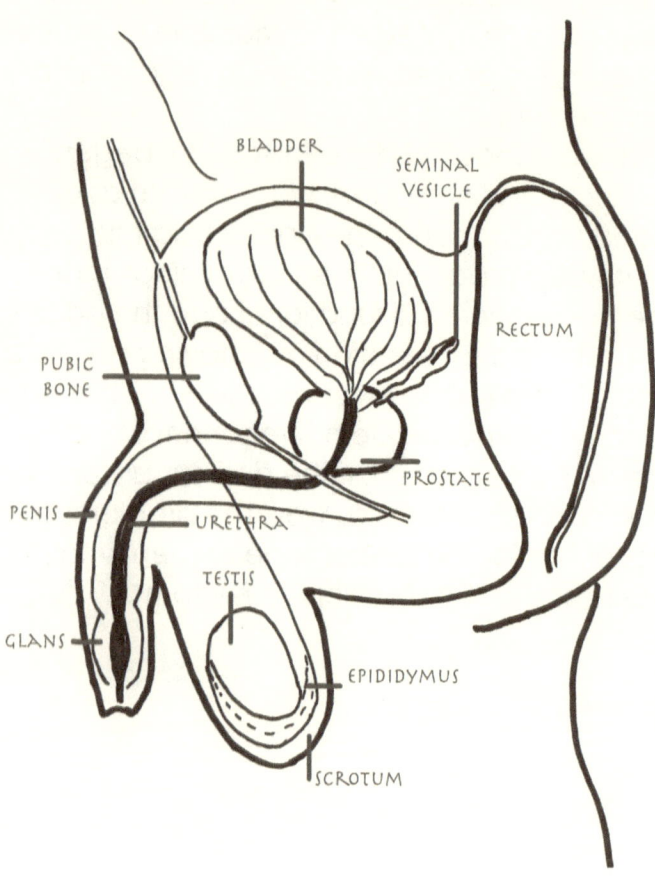

CHAPTER 7

SEX

I will remind the reader that this book reflects the personal experiences of my husband and myself. Every couple copes differently and every experience is unique. I approached sex following Gerry's surgery with the mindset that whatever challenges were thrown at us would be met with an open mind, humor and the goal of a full and satisfying sex life at the end of the healing process. It did take time, effort and humor, but the goal of mutual sexual satisfaction has been realized and I am confident that the end result was indeed a result of our willingness to experiment and to make the most of each encounter.

Sex is different after a radical prostatectomy. Period. No matter whom you ask. The seminal vesicles[8], urethra and bladder were

___

8 see pages 57-61 (Definitions)

all connected through the prostate. Once the prostate has been removed, the pieces that all fed through the prostate must now connect directly. No more middle man. The body must adapt to the changes necessitated by removal of the prostate.

Not all surgeons are equal. Not all patient's bodies will adapt equally. Some surgeons are better skilled. My surgeon father-in-law used to say that in the practice of surgery, numbers count. The more surgeries a doctor performs, the more skilled they become. This is true for traditional surgery as well as laser surgery aided by the daVinci© machine. The better the skill of the surgeon, the better the chance at nerve preservation and successful bodily functions.

I sought guidance from Dr. Jackson over the course of several years post-surgery about what to expect sexually and asked what we could do to improve our experience. Dr. Jackson was evasive. He was reluctant to provide concrete expectations or specific ways to work through the sexual part of recovery. I had expected a physician whose specialty included a great percentage of men with erectile dysfunction to be more helpful. I believed that a person who carefully maintained statistics on sexual recovery from surgery would be in a position to offer advice.

The one useful comment that I recall came many months after the surgery. As Gerry recovered and regained more control over the incontinence, Dr. Jackson suggested purchasing a pump to assist in gaining a functional erection and at the same time prescribed erectile dysfunction pills.

Dr. Jackson recommended that Gerry keep the pump in the bathroom and use it several times a week before his shower. We didn't understand the purpose of this exercise, so we asked. The explanation given was that the pump exercised the sacks that engorge the penis with blood. He said that the capability to have an erection would atrophy if not exercised. The more a muscle is used, the better it performs. I don't know why we didn't take that one bit of offered advice to heart, but we now believe that if Gerry had used the pump on a regular schedule, his sexual performance level would have improved sooner.

We looked at the different pump device models on the Internet and chose a battery-operated style. The range of choices and prices vary widely. It is important to note that the medical device is different than what is sold as a sex aid. The important component of the pump is the correct size band. Most models include a variety of band sizes so you don't have to guess when ordering. The model that we purchased was reasonably priced and proved to be easy to use and easy to clean. The pump arrived with a video showing how to use it properly. It still works and we still use it today, years later.

The first sexual encounter for Gerry and I was shortly after the catheter was removed. As I was waking one morning, I became aware of Gerry pressing his groin against my buttocks in his sleep. Prior to surgery, he often wakened with an erection and some mornings I would guide his penis inside of me and wake him up in the nicest way.

The feeling was the same, but instead of a rigid erection, the penis pushing against me felt more like a hot little bump. I turned over and placed his penis in my hand. It was small, not more than a little nub, yet firm. I could tell that it was an erection, regardless of the size. Immediately I began to stroke it, paying special attention to the head, knowing that it is the most sensitive part of the organ. Gerry groaned and wakened slowly. He looked at me and said, "My God, that feels so good." We lay in bed kissing and stroking each other toward orgasm. As Gerry became more excited, urine began a steady stream from his penis. As he reached climax, the urine was flowing freely.

We were soaked in urine, but ecstatic about the orgasm. So what if Gerry's penis was the size of a peanut. This was proof that his nerves were still viable. He had his first "erection" and was able to achieve orgasm. If I had missed this early opportunity, who knows how long it would have been before we figured out that he could climax, even without a visible erection? This was our first lesson that sex would need to be redefined and confirmation the urethra was now connected directly to the bladder.

Fortunately, we had already covered the mattress with a waterproof pad. I washed all of our bedding and heaped our inventory of thick, absorbent towels at the foot of the bed. Now I knew we could work on our new sex life. Knew that it would be messy. Knew that an erection of some kind was possible, but had no idea if Gerry would ever have a fully functional penis that would allow vaginal penetration or if we would be able to have sex without pee.

We continued to experiment. Fortunately neither of us is squeamish. Foreplay became a much bigger deal than before. Gerry and I would prepare the bed, pile on towels, and warm a tube of KY jelly in the microwave and play. We discovered new secrets to each other's bodies. By nature, men are turned on visually, but after surgery I realized that Gerry responded to touch more than before. Other men have told me that they are more turned on by physical contact following their prostatectomy. We would start out by lying on our side, kissing and gently touching.

When I felt Gerry beginning to move and the urine begin to drip I would slide down his body, take his still small, drippy penis into my mouth and suck. It took some adjusting. I did not want to swallow urine; I let it escape from the side of my mouth. I did not want Gerry to feel self-conscious. Instead of being made aware of the leakage, he simply responded to the pleasure of oral sex.

Sometimes I would climb on top and we would mutually gratify each other orally. In the early days after surgery, I always crawled on top so that I would not accidently swallow urine. I wanted to be able to direct the leakage to the towel. Other times, I would simply open my legs wide and he would bring me to orgasm manually. He would very gently make small circles around and on the small nub at the top of my clitoris. As I became wet, he would also insert fingers inside my vagina while continuing the lazy circles around my clitoris using his thumb. This method was successful every time.

Another position that was effective in our early period of experimentation was for Gerry to sit on his knees, balanced on his heels. This gave me complete access to his penis and testicles. I would lie on my side with my bottom leg bent and my top leg positioned so that I was wide open for him, my head squarely between his legs. This position gave him total access to my body; he could manipulate my breasts, stroke my clitoris and insert his fingers into my vagina while I performed fellatio and gently played with his testicles. This position placed my head so that I could easily let the urine drain from my mouth without making him aware of it.

The early stages of sexual recovery were made much easier by finding creative ways of mutual satisfaction. Of course we missed quickies and impulsive sex. I missed the sensations that can only be felt by the deep penetration achieved by a hard, throbbing penis with the full thrusting weight of a man. I know Gerry missed it too. Sex toys were not satisfying to me, but they are a readily available option and many people find them stimulating and an exciting addition to sex play.

One sunny day we found ourselves alone, at home with no obligations. I had been outside gardening and when I came in for a shower, Gerry hopped in too. We have always showered together, but that day as we were cleaning up, I was poked in the belly by a distinctly erect penis. Excited, I shouted, "Look, look, Gerry, you have an erection. A real one." Whoo hoo-we grabbed our towels and ran to the bed. I couldn't believe it. This was the first time that I had seen his penis completely erect, engorged and looking like it used to. All without drugs or appliances. We sat face-to-face on the bed, his penis hard enough for me to sit on top and reveled in our first unplanned sexual encounter. It was exciting and immensely satisfying.

Our excitement abated as days and weeks passed without another spontaneous erection, but we were encouraged to work harder because now we knew for certain that "normal" sex was possible.

Over time we learned that sunlight enhanced Gerry's libido and we arranged our days as much as possible to allow time for sex during the day. Sex was still time consuming, due to medication constraints.

Gerry experimented with Viagra, Cialis and Levitra. Unfortunately, he experienced almost all of the listed side effects with all of the drugs. Skin flushing, headache, blue vision, lightheadedness. Gerry's erections were improved when he used pills, but using them reduced his ability to function for the remainder of the day. We learned to take that into account. If he had to return to work, or think clearly afterwards, he would skip the pill and rely on the pump exclusively. As Gerry regained urinary continence, the urine flow during sex decreased accordingly.

A positive aspect of a prostatectomy for some women is that orgasms no longer produce semen. If a woman doesn't like to have a man come in her mouth, it's no longer an issue. When the urine drip ceases, oral sex is no longer a messy proposition.

Hopefully this will help women who find semen objectionable enjoy oral sex in a more relaxed way. If a couple is not used to having oral sex, this surgery is a perfect time to start. Immediately after surgery, the penis is not as large or erect as before, so concerns about choking are alleviated. By the time the penis becomes fully erect again, it should be exciting, not scary or gross. It's a great time to experiment and learn what feels good to both parties.

There was a stage for Gerry, when aroused; his penis became erect, but not yet hard. It was frustrating, because we just wanted good hard sex, but penetration wasn't possible; or so we thought. We were wrong.

Through experimentation, we found that even if the erection isn't firm, penetration can be achieved by rear entry. If I propped myself doggy style, my rear-end in the air, Gerry was able to enter and thrust to orgasm. We found other rear-entry positions. I could bend over the back of a chair or sofa allowing easy rear entry. I could kneel on the edge of the bed, with Gerry standing behind me, holding my hips and thrusting. By adapting we were able to have spontaneous sex again.

My new favorite position does require a full erection, which can be achieved with the help of a pump, or pill, or combination, if needed. This position allows for the deepest penetration and feels insanely good to both of us. I lie curled on my side. Legs bent. Gerry gets on his knees, body upright, at the bend of my knees. He enters me from the side. This position makes use of his full weight, without crushing me and achieves complete penetration. I love it when he flips me on to my side and enters me this way. It satisfies me completely and judging from Gerry's response to me, he loves it every bit as much as I do.

CHAPTER 8

CONCLUSION

This book is not a recommendation for or against any type of medical treatment. Only your doctor can advise and recommend appropriate treatment for your particular circumstance.

This is a personal chronicle, detailing the experience of my husband and myself. There were stages throughout our experience that were profoundly frustrating for me and this is exactly the type of book that I had searched for after Gerry's diagnosis of prostate cancer.

All opinions expressed are mine alone. Names have been changed to protect and respect the privacy of others.

———

Gerry and I have had more challenges over the past five years than I would have believed possible. Our middle years find us starting over in several major facets of life.

Gerry's illness arrived simultaneously at a critical time for our business. We were in the midst of merger negotiations and had just spent several years completing the R&D phase of a large project. The distraction of prostate cancer treatment combined with the economic downturn strained our financial resources to the brink. We were broke. We were faced with yet another life-altering decision to make.

Prostate cancer caused us to reevaluate our priorities. We made the decision to close the business, an institution that until this moment had been the center of our lives. We chose to spend our remaining years focused on family. Our needs are modest. We want time, not stuff. We must find a way to meet our paired-down financial needs without compromising our priority of time together.

Gerry has chosen a career path that he is very excited about. He enrolled in a local college, completing a degree in a profession that is completely different from our prior field of expertise. I have worked in the medical field in the interim to cover our basic expenses.

My position places me in direct contact with men who are dealing with prostate cancer and asking the same questions that Gerry and I had. Hearing the concerns and fears of these men as they come to terms with prostate cancer and struggle with the difficulties of treatment confirms my observation that other couples might benefit from my experience as the wife of a man struggling to recover his sexual prowess after removal of his prostate.

Our experience with prostate cancer has been a blessing-in-disguise. Being forced to focus our energy on a very intimate and frightening disease has strengthened our marriage and commitment to each other.

Gerry and I are grateful that prostate cancer has not prevented our ability to move forward. We are grateful to have found ways to sustain intimacy and have a fully satisfying sexual life.

We look forward to completing our journey, wherever it may lead, together.

We begin anew.

I wish the same for you.

DEFINITIONS

<u>ANUS</u>- Opening for release of feces
<u>BLADDER</u>- Sac that contains urine
<u>EPIDIDYMUS</u>-The tube that contains sperm
<u>GLEASON SCORE-</u>A diagnostic tool for rating prostate cancer is called the "Gleason Score". I had never heard this term before Gerry's

As explained to us: Multiple biopsy samples often show varying degrees of cancer (another reason to have as many samples to review as possible, because it can be hit or miss)

This was all very confusing to me and I have attempted to break it down, but it is imperative that you to talk to your doctor until you clearly understand how these numbers relate to your specific cancer.

<u>Grading:</u> The Primary Gleason Grade has to be greater than 50% of the total cancer seen and the Secondary Gleason Grade (must be less

than 50%, but at least 5%, of the pattern of the total cancer seen)
Primary grade + Secondary grade = GS
Examples:

- 3+5=8
- 5+3=8

In the first example, the primary Gleason Grade=3. That means that the primary cancer found is low risk. The second example, the primary Gleason Grade=5. That means that the primary cancer found is considered moderately aggressive. Both examples total 8, but where the numbers are located dictate how the cancer will be treated.

Gleason Score: (GS) is the sum of the primary grade and the secondary grade.
The higher the Gleason score, the more aggressive the tumor is likely to act and the worse the patient's prognosis.

The cancer aggression scale reads like this:
A total GS of 2 to 4 are considered low on the cancer aggression scale.
A total GS of 5-6 are considered mildly aggressive.
A total GS of 7 indicates that the cancer is moderately aggressive
A total of 8-10 indicates a highly aggressive cancer

<u>PENIS</u>-Male sex organ

<u>PROSTATE</u>-The prostate is a small, squishy gland that sits under the bladder and in front of the rectum. Running alongside and attached to the sides of the prostate are the nerves that control erectile function.

<u>PSA TEST/ANNUAL EXAM</u>-As a matter of course, men and women have different reproductive organs and annual physical exams reflect those differentials. A routine exam for either sex will include a basic blood panel. There are additional tests performed that are specific to one's sex. An annual "complete physical" or "wellness visit" for a man the age of 40+ should include checking testosterone levels as well as a PSA test and a rectal exam.

The PSA (Prostate Specific Antigen) test is a simple blood test. Healthy men have low PSA present in the blood stream. An enlarging prostate is part of the aging process and the PSA present in the blood will increase accordingly. Other reasons for an increase of the PSA number could indicate inflammation of or prostate cancer. A PSA test alone does not diagnose prostate cancer.

If the blood test shows an elevated PSA number, the physician may choose to re-test at a later time, or he or she could recommend a biopsy. The recommendation will be based on your doctor's knowledge of your personal family history as well as his or her medical experience.

The rectal exam should also be a component of the routine physical. It is an additional way to examine the prostate. While it may be slightly embarrassing or uncomfortable for some men, others aren't bothered at all. Either way, it is an important diagnostic tool.

The process is very straightforward. The physician inserts a gloved finger into the rectum where he has direct access to the prostate gland-he can then feel for enlargement of the prostate and hard lumps that could be an early indicator of a tumor. This important step can detect the first signs of trouble particularly if the man is too young for routine PSA screening, and therefore, should not be omitted.

Symptoms of frequent urination, difficulty holding urine stream, difficulty starting urination, frequent pain or stiffness in the lower back, hips or upper thighs, difficulty having an erection or painful ejaculation, should be reported to your doctor. These symptoms could be indicative of an elevated PSA or other undiagnosed condition.

RISK CATEGORIES
A.   Age - Age is the strongest risk factor for prostate cancer. Prostate cancer is unusual before the age of 40, but the chance of having prostate cancer increases rapidly after age 50
B.   Race/Ethnicity - African-American men are in the highest risk category, followed by Caucasians. Asian, Hispanic and Native American's have the lowest risk.

C.   <u>Nationality</u> - Prostate cancer is most common in North America, Northwestern Europe, Australia and in the Caribbean.

D.   <u>Family History</u> - Having a father or brother with prostate cancer increases the risk of developing this disease.

F.   <u>Diet</u> – It is possible that men who eat a lot of red meat and high fat dairy products are at greater risk and men whose diets are rich in vegetables, fruit, whole grains, poultry and fish are at a lower risk.

<u>SCROTUM</u>-The pouch containing testicles
<u>SEMINAL VESICLES</u>-Glands located on each side of the bladder that secretes seminal fluid and pushes the sperm from beginning to end.
<u>TESTIS</u>-The organ that produces sperm
<u>URETHRA</u>- The tube through which urine flows, running through the prostate and penis
<u>VAS DEFERENS</u>-Tube connecting the testes with the urethra

RESOURCES

http://www.dummies.com/how-to/content/
making-the-grade-with-the-gleason-score.html
www.ustoo.org
http://www.pcf.org/site/c.leJRIROrEpH/
b.5699537/k.BEF4/Home.htm
http://www.cancer.gov/cancertopics/types/
prostate
http://www.urologychannel.com/prostatecan-
cer/treatment-surg.shtml
http://health.nytimes.com/health/guides/dis-
ease/prostate-cancer
http://health.usnews.com/usnews/health/
articles/070909/17prostate.htm
http://www.mayoclinic.com/health/cancer/
CA00049
http://www.medicalnewstoday.com/arti-
cles/84936.php

www.ingramcontent.com/pod-product-compliance
Lightning Source LLC
Chambersburg PA
CBHW021237280526
45784CB00005B/2133